ACID REFLUX REVERSAL MANUAL AND COOKBOOK

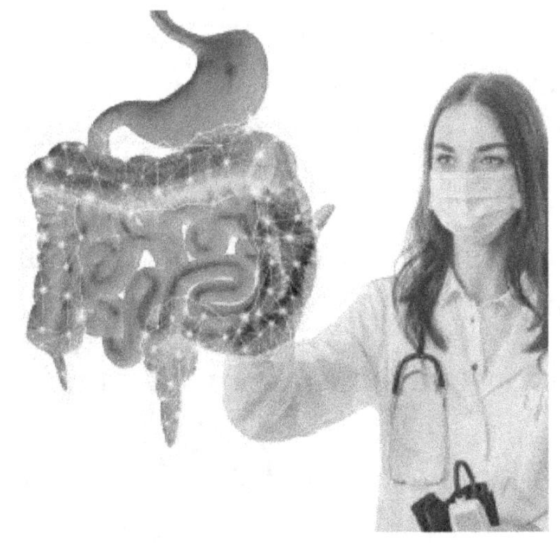

A Comprehensive Guide to Managing Acid Reflux and Quick and Easy Delicious Recipes to Combat GERD, LPR, and Heartburns.

Mary D. Johnson

Acid Reflux Reversal Manual and Cookbook

Copyright © 2024 [Mary D. Johnson]

For permission requests, write to the publisher at the address below:

[mary.d.johnsonhelpdesk@gmail.com]

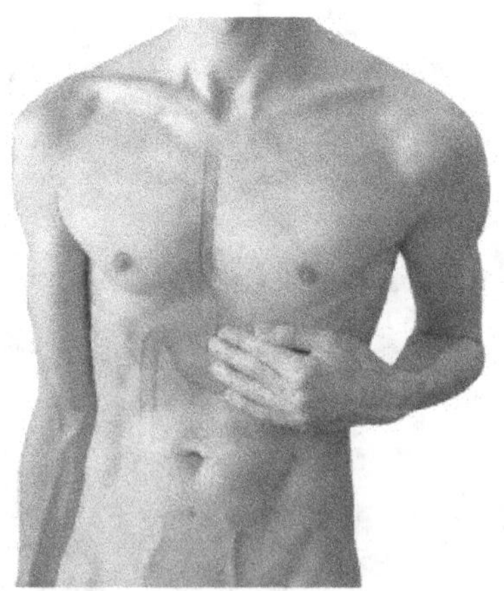

TABLE OF CONTENTS

I.   INTRODUCTION

Do you often experience a burning sensation in the chest or throat, especially after eating, bending over, or lying down? Have you ever had a disrupted sleep during nighttime due to this fiery discomfort and intense pressure? If you ever had one, this condition is not peculiar to you. Millions of people around the world suffering from acid reflux experience similar or even worse symptoms including Helen, whose condition brought her into contact with me.

Helen's story echoes the struggles of countless individuals who have battled the relentless discomfort brought on by acid reflux. The persistent burning sensation, the uneasy feeling after each meal, and the nagging pain that became a constant companion – these were the challenges Helen faced daily. It's a story that may sound familiar to you or someone you know, as acid reflux affects millions worldwide.

Imagine sitting down to savor a delicious meal, only to be interrupted by the unwelcome surge of acid into your esophagus. Helen knows this all too well. For years, she sought relief through various medications, hoping for that elusive moment of respite. Yet, the relief she craved remained just out of reach. It was in the midst of this struggle that she found her way to a different path – one that would ultimately lead her to a life free from the grips of acid reflux.

I vividly remember the day Helen walked into my life. A mutual friend, concerned for her well-being, introduced us. Helen was at her wits' end, tired of the constant discomfort that seemed to define her existence. The medications she had relied on provided only fleeting relief, leaving her desperate for a more sustainable solution.

As we sat down over tea, Helen shared her journey with me. The frustration, the sleepless nights, and the toll it had taken on her overall well-being were palpable in her words. It was a story that resonated deeply with me, as I had witnessed similar struggles in many others I had encountered over the years.

Armed with a determination to bring about positive change, Helen decided to embark on a journey of healing through a tailored diet regimen I recommended. She took a leap of faith, choosing a path less traveled but filled with the promise of relief. She did not realize at first that this decision would signal the beginning of her journey to healthy living.

The journey to acid reflux reversal is not just about dietary changes; it's a holistic approach that addresses the root causes of the issue. It's about understanding the nuances of our bodies, the impact of our choices, and the power we hold to shape our well-being. Helen embraced this philosophy wholeheartedly, diving into the recommended dietary adjustments with a newfound hope.

As she navigated the landscape of acid reflux-friendly foods, incorporating flavorful yet soothing recipes into her daily routine, Helen began to experience a gradual shift. The burning sensation that had once been a constant presence started to fade. The uneasy feeling after meals was replaced by a sense of satisfaction, and the nagging pain became a distant memory.

It wasn't an overnight transformation, but a journey of consistent choices and mindful eating. Helen's dedication to the recommended diet regimen became a testament to the incredible resilience of the human body and its capacity to heal when provided with the right tools.

Today, as Helen looks back on her journey, she marvels at the profound impact these dietary changes have had on her life. No longer defined by the discomfort of acid reflux, she has reclaimed the joy of sharing meals with loved ones and savoring the simple pleasures of life. Her story serves as a beacon of hope for those who, like her, have yearned for a way out of the cycle of acid reflux.

In this cookbook, I invite you to join me on a journey – a journey to discover the art of crafting meals that not only delight the taste buds but also promote digestive health. Together, we'll explore the meaning and intricacies of acid reflux, unraveling its causes and symptoms. We'll delve into practical strategies for prevention and management, understanding the importance of both what to embrace and what to avoid.

But this book is not just a collection of information; it's a guide infused with the personal touch of individuals who have triumphed over acid reflux. Helen's story is just one among many, and as you navigate through these pages, you'll encounter real-world examples, relatable anecdotes, and a wealth of recipes designed to make your journey to acid reflux reversal not only effective but also enjoyable.

So, grab a cup of tea or coffee, get comfortable, and let's embark on this journey together. From heartburn to happiness – it's a path that's possible and within your reach. Welcome to a life where meals are not a source of discomfort but a celebration of well-being.

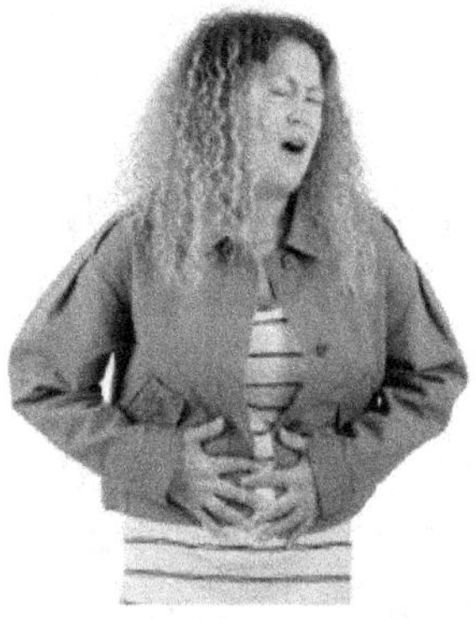

Acid reflux patient

II. Understanding Acid Reflux

CHAPTER 1: WHAT IS ACID REFLUX?

Acid reflux is like a gentle whisper that goes unheard until it becomes a clamorous presence in our daily lives. It's caused by stomach acid traveling uninvitedly back into the esophagus, causing pain ranging from a burning feeling to regurgitation. To grasp this phenomenon, let us dig into the deep aspects of acid reflux and distinguish between its numerous manifestations.

The Heart of Acid Reflux

Acid reflux occurs when the lower esophageal sphincter, a muscle valve that separates the stomach from the esophagus, fails to operate correctly. This flaw permits stomach acid to travel backward, resulting in various acid reflux symptoms.

Types of Acid Reflux
Gastroesophageal Reflux Disease (GERD):

Chronic and Persistent: GERD, as opposed to occasional heartburn, is a chronic illness characterized by frequent acid reflux.

Underlying difficulties: GERD is frequently caused by underlying difficulties such as a weakening lower esophageal sphincter, obesity, a hiatal hernia, pregnancy, or the use of certain drugs.

Silent Nature: GERD may be sneaky, manifesting itself through symptoms such as persistent cough, hoarseness, or tooth issues making it critical to treat not only the symptoms but the underlying causes as well.

Heartburn:

Occasional and fleeting: Heartburn is an occasional guest in the realm of acid reflux.

Triggered by Lifestyle or Foods: It is frequently caused by certain foods or lifestyle practices that temporarily relax the lower esophageal sphincter.

Quick Departure: Heartburn, unlike GERD, tends to disappear soon after the triggering event.

Acid Regurgitation:

Backward Flow of Acid: This kind is distinguished by the regurgitation of stomach acid into the esophagus.

Common Symptom: Acid regurgitation is frequently combined with additional symptoms, adding to the total pain associated with acid reflux.

Deciphering the Discomfort Language

Understanding acid reflux is like deciphering the language of suffering. It all starts with the lower esophageal sphincter, a key role in maintaining the balance between the stomach and the esophagus. When this muscle valve fails, stomach acid returns, causing the typical burning feeling and disquiet.

The Culprits Within

A disruption in the function of the lower esophageal sphincter can be caused by several factors. Obesity, a hiatal hernia, pregnancy, or the use of particular drugs all contribute to miscommunication within our digestive system, causing acid to infiltrate where it doesn't belong.

The Symphony of Symptoms

Acid reflux is a symphony of symptoms people may experience in various combinations. Acid reflux symptoms range from conventional heartburn to regurgitation, chest pain, and even a chronic cough.

We've covered the basics of acid reflux, distinguishing between its chronic form, GERD, and the more transient heartburn. Understanding this language of discomfort is the first step in breaking free from the grip of acid reflux. As we progress through the chapters, we'll look not just at the complexities of its language, but also at practical ways of decoding and managing it efficiently. Join me as we traverse this route together, arming ourselves with the information we need to reclaim a life free of the challenges of acid reflux.

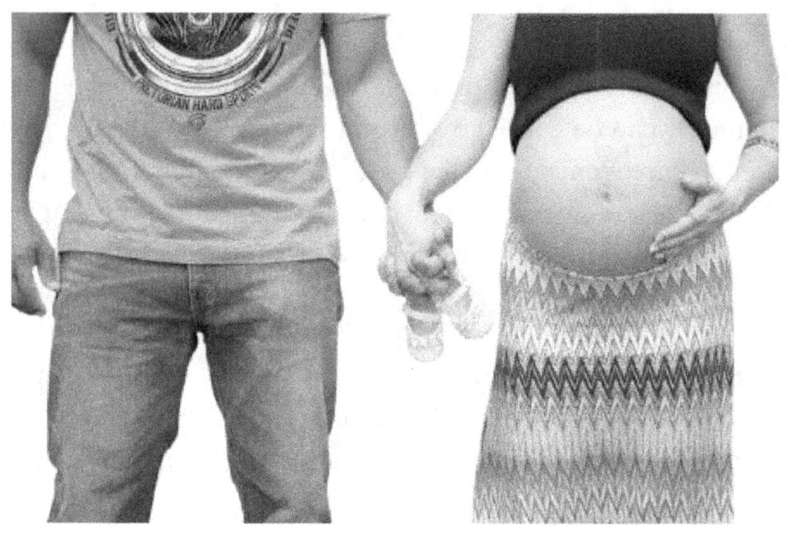

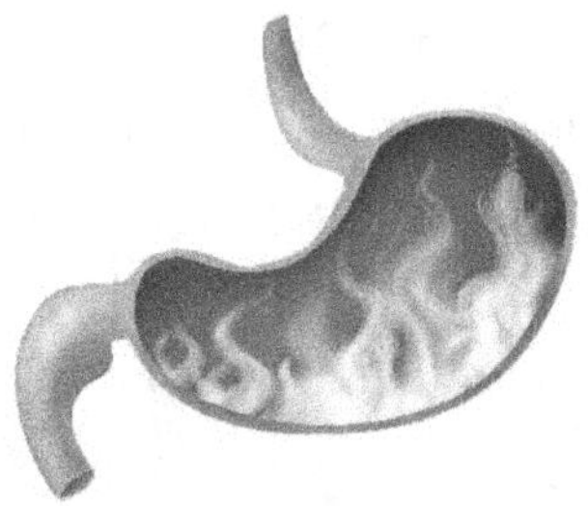

HEARTBURN

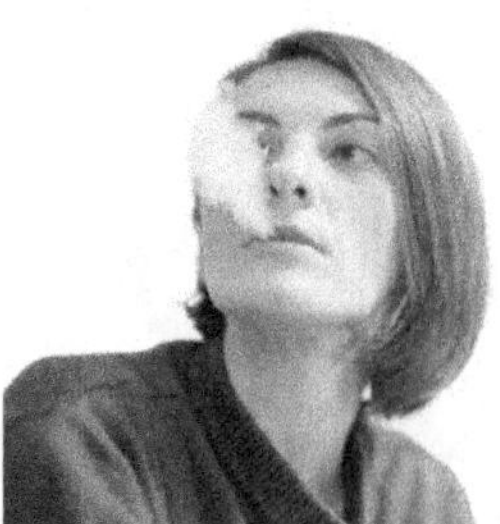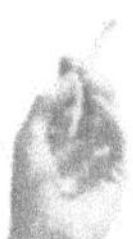

CHAPTER 2: COMMON CAUSES OF ACID REFLUX

Understanding the causes of acid reflux is essential for navigating the path to relief and reversal. While it is commonly associated with overindulging in spicy or acidic foods, the triggers for acid reflux are diverse and can range from lifestyle choices to underlying health concerns.

Dietary Offenders

Fatty Foods: Consuming high-fat meals can significantly contribute to acid reflux. Fats impede digestion, enabling stomach contents to linger and increasing the incidence of reflux.

Citrus and tomato-based products: Citric acid, which is found in oranges, tomatoes, and their derivatives, is a known acid reflux trigger. These acidic substances might irritate the esophagus, exacerbating the pain.

Spicy Delights: While spice adds taste to our meals, it can also promote the formation of stomach acid, potentially leading to reflux. Spicy foods should be avoided if you suffer from acid reflux.

Lifestyle Factors

Overeating: Overeating puts undue strain on the lower esophageal sphincter, increasing the likelihood of stomach contents flowing back into the esophagus.

Late-night Snacking: Eating close to bedtime might slow digestion, increasing the risk of acid reflux during the night. Gravity is important in preventing reflux, and lying down too soon after eating undermines this natural barrier.

Smoking and Alcohol: Smoking and heavy alcohol use can both weaken the lower esophageal sphincter, increasing acid reflux. Furthermore, drinking might increase stomach acid production.

Physical Factors

Obesity: Obesity puts pressure on the abdomen, which can drive stomach acid into the esophagus. Obesity may be dramatically reduced by making lifestyle adjustments.

Hiatal Hernia: This happens when the top section of the stomach protrudes through the diaphragm into the chest cavity. Hiatal hernias can cause acid reflux by weakening the lower esophageal sphincter.

Pregnancy

Hormonal Changes: Pregnancy causes hormonal changes that loosen the lower esophageal sphincter, allowing for more acid reflux. The expanding uterus also puts pressure on the stomach.

Symptoms and Their Varieties

Acid reflux symptoms are as varied as its causes, making it critical to know the numerous ways it might manifest itself.

Heartburn: The characteristic symptom, characterized by a burning feeling in the chest. It frequently happens after meals and can be aggravated by reclining down.

Regurgitation: The backflow of stomach contents into the mouth, resulting in a sour or bitter taste. This is a very unpleasant symptom of acid reflux.

Chest Pain: While not necessarily as severe as a heart attack, chest pain can accompany acid reflux, creating discomfort and anxiety.

Chronic Cough: Acid reflux can irritate the throat, resulting in a persistent cough. This symptom is sometimes disregarded as a possible symptom of reflux.

Hoarseness: Stomach acid reaching the vocal cords can cause discomfort, resulting in hoarseness or a raspy voice.

Difficulty Swallowing: Acid reflux can cause a lump in the throat or difficulty swallowing in certain people, a condition known as dysphagia.

Sleep Disruptions: Acid reflux throughout the night can interrupt sleep, producing restless nights and adding to exhaustion.

Understanding the many causes and symptoms of acid reflux sets the groundwork for efficient therapy. As we proceed along this path, we'll learn more about tactics that not only relieve symptoms but also help to reverse the discomfort produced by acid reflux.

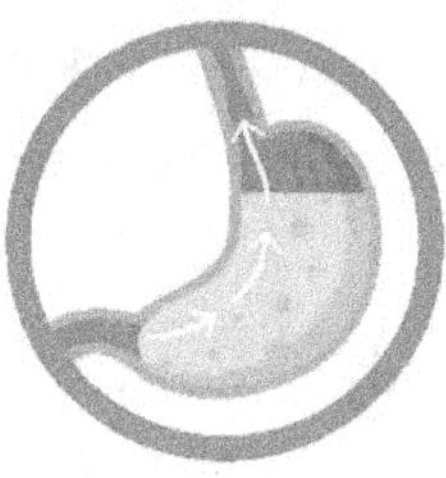

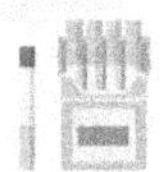
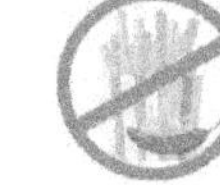
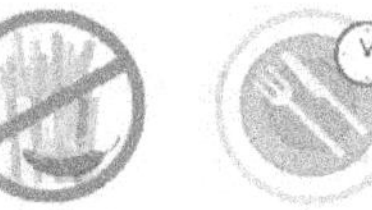

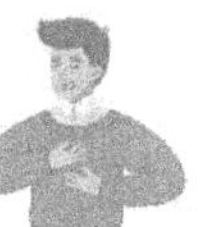
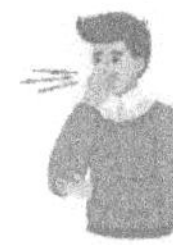
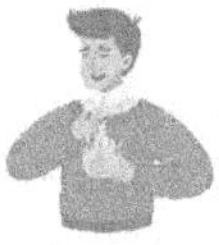
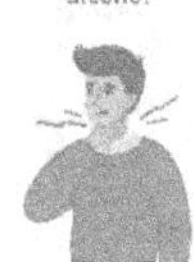

GASTROESOPHAGEAL REFLUX DISEASE
RISK FACTORS & SYMPTOMS

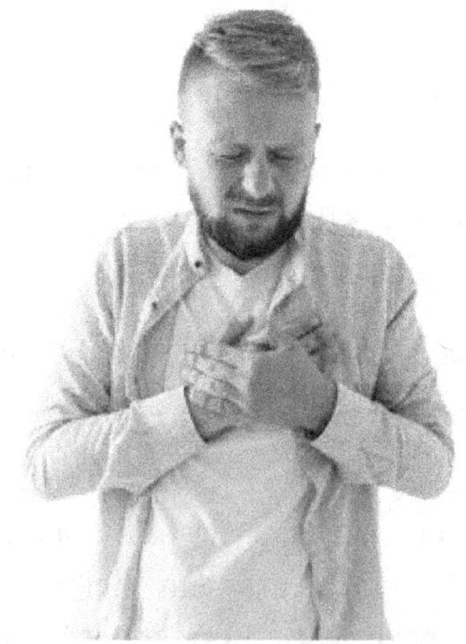

CHAPTER 3: ACID REFLUX RISK FACTORS

Certain risk variables emerge as crucial elements in the complicated tapestry of acid reflux, determining the frequency and severity of this prevalent condition. Understanding these aspects is critical in developing a tailored preventative and treatment approach.

1. Obesity: A Significant Contributor to Abdominal Pressure:

Excess weight, particularly around the belly, can put unnecessary strain on the stomach. This pressure creates an environment that allows stomach acid to move upward into the esophagus.

Increased Risk of Hiatal Hernia: Obesity is frequently connected to the development of hiatal hernias, further weakening the barrier between the stomach and the esophagus.

2. Hiatal Hernia: Bridging the Gap

Anatomical Shift: A hiatal hernia arises when a part of the stomach protrudes into the chest cavity via the diaphragm. This anatomical alteration undermines the integrity of the lower esophageal sphincter, allowing stomach contents to reflux.

Common in Older Adults: Hiatal hernias are more common in older persons, rendering older people more prone to acid reflux.

3. Hormonal Changes During Pregnancy

Lower Esophageal Sphincter Relaxation: Pregnancy causes hormonal changes, including the production of progesterone, which relaxes the lower esophageal sphincter. This relaxation adds to an increase in acid reflux among pregnant women.

Uterus Pressure: As the uterus grows to support the developing baby, it can put pressure on the stomach, increasing the risk of acid reflux.

4. Smoking:

Lower Esophageal Sphincter Weakening: Smoking weakens the lower esophageal sphincter, reducing its capacity to control the backward passage of stomach acid.

Reduced Saliva Production: Smoking reduces saliva production, which is important for neutralizing stomach acid. The decrease in saliva exacerbates the acidic environment in the esophagus.

5. Alcohol: A Double-Edged Sword

Relaxation of the Lower Esophageal Sphincter: Alcohol, like smoking, relaxes the lower esophageal sphincter, facilitating acid reflux.

Increased Acid Production: Alcohol causes the stomach to create more acid, increasing the likelihood of reflux.

6. Age: A Gradual Influence on Lower Esophageal Sphincter Tone:

As people become older, the tone of their lower esophageal sphincter gradually decreases, leaving them more prone to acid reflux.

Accumulation of Risk Factors: As people age, they may acquire more risk factors, such as obesity or hiatal hernias, which increases the incidence of acid reflux.

7. Medications: Adverse Effects on the Lower Esophageal Sphincter

Certain drugs, such as antihypertensives, sedatives, and calcium channel blockers, can relax the lower esophageal sphincter, allowing acid reflux to occur.

Direct Irritation: Some drugs may cause direct esophageal irritation, contributing to the development or worsening of acid reflux symptoms.

8. Delayed Stomach Emptying:

The Prolonged Pause Impairs Digestive Process: Acid reflux can be exacerbated by conditions that cause delayed stomach emptying, such as gastroparesis. When the stomach takes longer to empty, the possibility of reflux increases.

9. Dietary Choices: What You Eat Is Important

High-Fat Diets: Fat-rich diets can impede digestion, extending the presence of food in the stomach and raising the likelihood of reflux.

Acidic and spicy foods: Tomatoes, citrus fruits, and spicy food can directly irritate the esophagus, causing acid reflux.

We've looked at the many risk factors that contribute to the development and worsening of acid reflux in this chapter. Recognizing these characteristics is an important first step in taking a proactive approach to treating this problem. As we move through this book, we'll look at techniques for mitigating these risks and empowering people to retake control over their gut health.

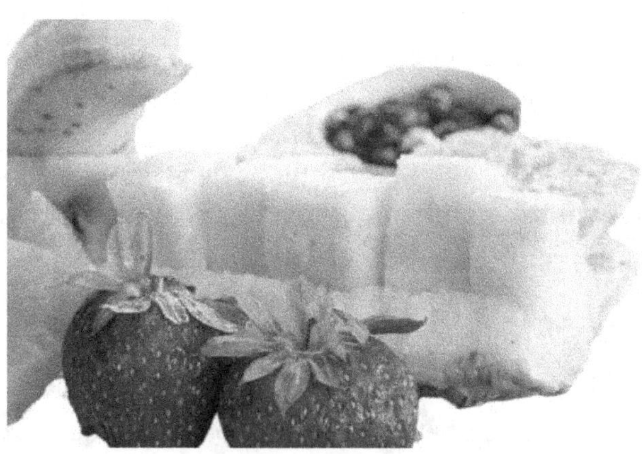

III. Taking Control: Prevention and Management

CHAPTER 4:

STRATEGIES FOR PREVENTION

Acid reflux disease (GERD) occurs when stomach acid runs back into the esophagus, producing irritation and discomfort. While drugs might give temporary relief, preventative efforts generally emphasize lifestyle modifications and the maintenance of digestive system health.

Here are key aspects to consider:

Lifestyle Changes to Prevent Acid Reflux

1. Dietary Changes:

• **Avoid Trigger Foods**: Certain foods, such as citrus fruits, tomatoes, chocolate, mint, garlic, onions, and spicy or fatty foods, can aggravate acid reflux.

• **Moderate Meal Size:** Eating smaller, more frequent meals might help reduce stomach overburden, lowering the chance of acid reflux.

• **Avoid Caffeine and Alcohol:** Caffeine and alcohol both relax the lower esophageal sphincter, which contributes to acid reflux. It is best to limit their consumption.

2.   Positional Changes:

• **Elevate the Head of the Bed:** Raising the head of the bed by 6 to 8 inches can help prevent stomach acid from flowing into the esophagus during sleep.

• **Avoid Lying Down Immediately After Meals:** Staying upright for two to three hours after eating will help digestion and lessen the risk of acid reflux.

• **Maintain a Healthy Weight:** Excess weight, particularly around the belly, can put a strain on the stomach which promotes acid reflux. Weight loss with a healthy diet and regular exercise can be beneficial.

4. Quit Smoking:

Nicotine in cigarettes can weaken the lower esophageal sphincter, enabling stomach acid to seep back into the esophagus. Giving up smoking is essential for general health and acid reflux prevention.

Tips for Keeping Your Digestive System Healthy:

1. Keep Hydrated:

• **Adequate Water Intake:** Drinking adequate water helps to maintain the mucosal lining of the esophagus, minimizing stomach acid discomfort.

• **Avoid Excessive Carbonated Beverages:** Carbonated beverages can cause bloating and raise stomach pressure, potentially leading to acid reflux.

2. Chew Food Properly:

• **Encourage Proper Digestion:** Chewing food properly assists in digestion, reducing the burden on the stomach and lowering the risk of acid reflux.

3. Regular Exercise:

• **Promotes Healthy Digestion:** Regular physical exercise regulates bowel motions and enhances overall digestive health.

• **Avoid Vigorous Exercise Just After Meals:** Vigorous exercise just after eating might increase the probability of acid reflux. Workouts should be scheduled at least a couple of hours after eating.

4. Manage Stress:

• **Mind-Body Techniques:** Practices like deep breathing, meditation, and yoga can help manage stress, which can contribute to digestive problems.

• **Establish Consistent Meal intervals:** Eating at regular intervals helps control digestion and can lessen the risk of acid reflux.

To summarize, acid reflux prevention is a mix of lifestyle adjustments and keeping a healthy digestive system.

Preventing acid reflux requires dietary modifications, positional changes, weight control, and quitting smoking. Furthermore, staying hydrated, chewing food properly, exercising regularly, and controlling stress all contribute to overall digestive health. Individuals can lessen the frequency and severity of acid reflux symptoms by using these preventive techniques, encouraging improved digestive health.

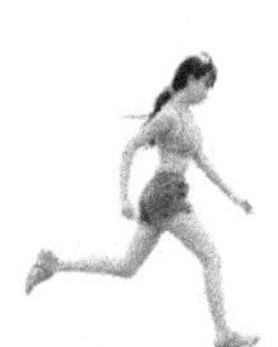

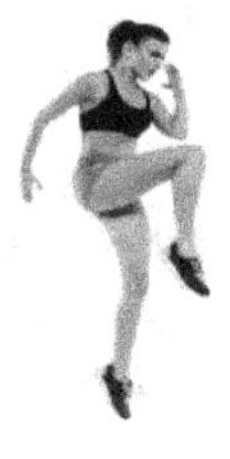

CHAPTER 5: FOODS TO AVOID

Acid reflux, also known as gastroesophageal reflux disease (GERD), is frequently impacted by dietary choices. It is essential to understand which foods to avoid to prevent or manage acid reflux. Here is a list of foods that may cause acid reflux, as well as an explanation of why they are problematic:

Foods that may trigger acid reflux include:

1. Citrus Fruits:

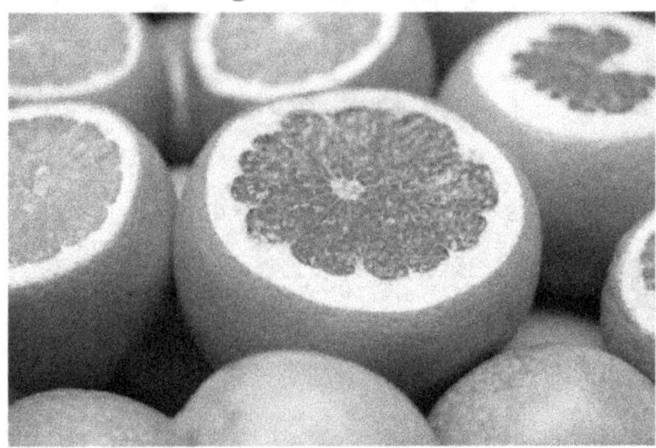

• Oranges, lemons, grapefruits, and other citrus fruits are acidic and might contribute to increased stomach acid, perhaps causing esophageal discomfort.

2. Tomatoes:

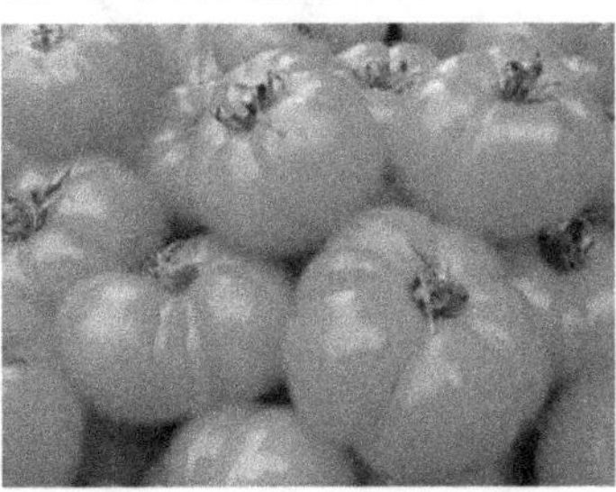

• Tomatoes and tomato-based products have significant amounts of acidity, which can cause the lower esophageal sphincter (LES) to relax, enabling stomach acid to flow into the esophagus.

3. Chocolate:

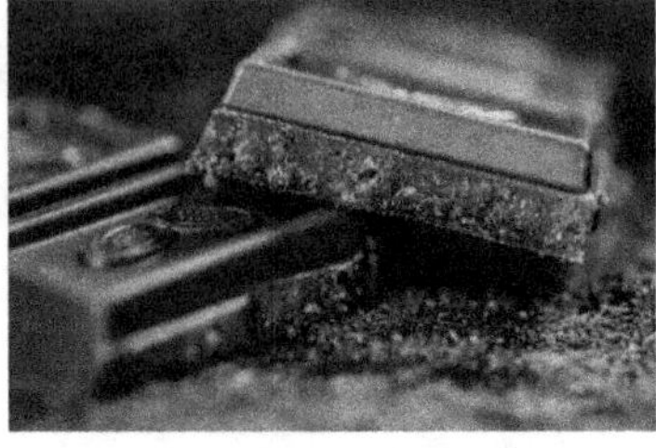

• Chocolate contains both caffeine and fat, which can both relax the LES. Furthermore, chocolate contains theobromine, a chemical that may aggravate acid reflux symptoms.

4. Mint:

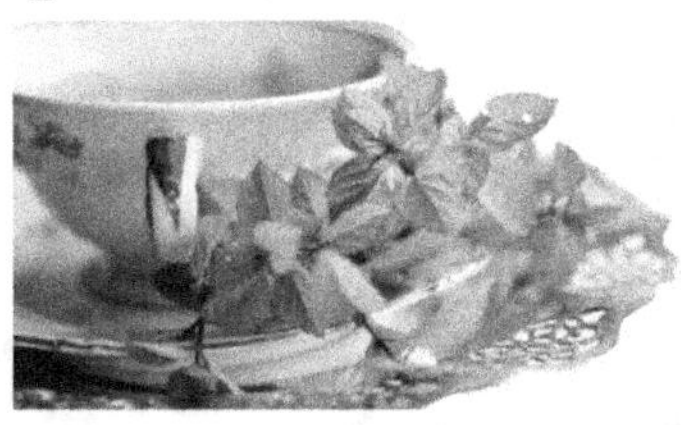

• Peppermint and spearmint, which are prominent in gums, candies, and teas, might relax the LES, resulting in increased acid reflux. Mint-flavored items may also add to the problems.

5. Onions and Garlic:

• Onions and garlic might promote LES relaxation and increase stomach acid production, thereby worsening acid reflux symptoms.

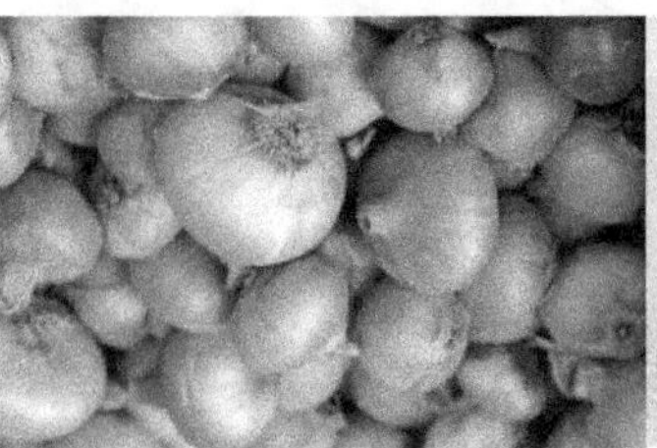 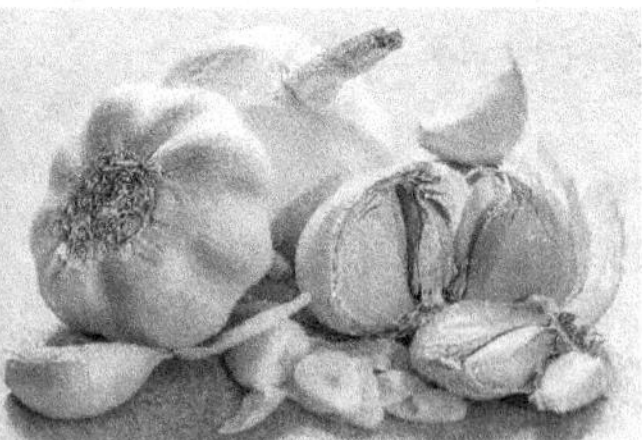

6. Spicy Foods:

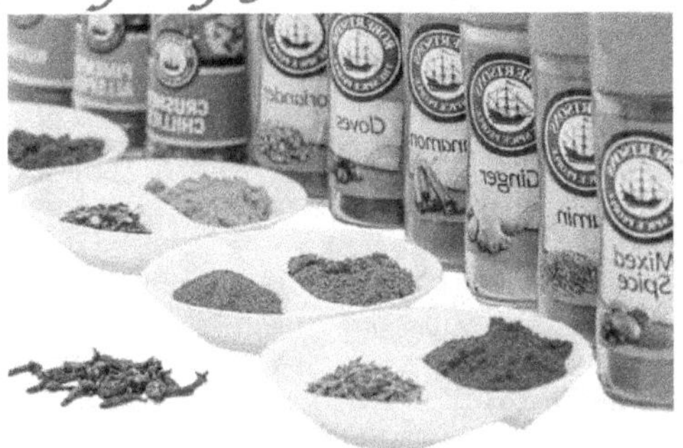

• Spices and spicy foods, such as chili peppers, can irritate the esophagus and induce acid reflux in those with allergies.

7. Fatty Foods:

• High-fat foods, such as fried foods, full-fat dairy products, and fatty meats, might delay stomach emptying and relax the LES, resulting in increased acid reflux.

8. Coffee and Caffeinated Beverages:

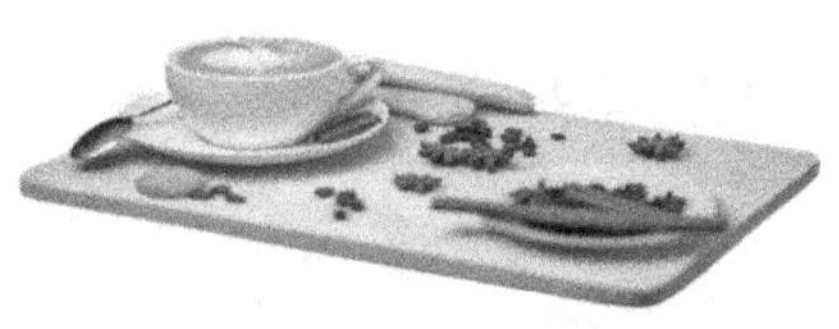

• Caffeine is known to relax the LES, allowing stomach acid to flow back into the esophagus. Caffeine is commonly found in coffee, tea, and some soft drinks.

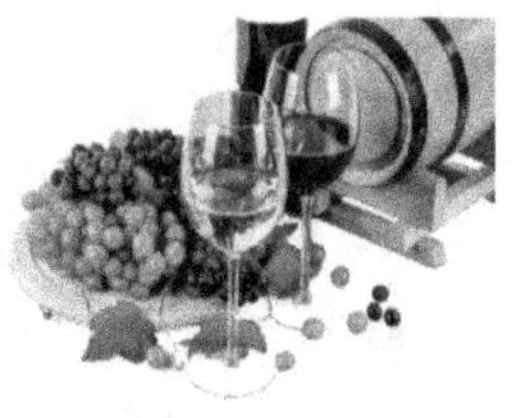

9. Alcohol:

• Alcohol can relax the LES and lead to increased stomach acid production, making it a possible acid reflux trigger.

10. Carbonated Beverages:

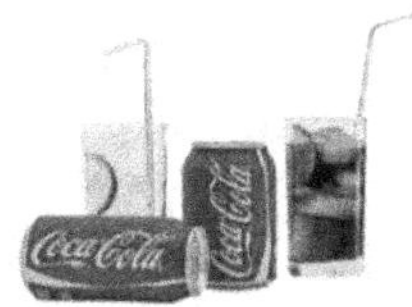

• Carbonated beverages, such as sodas and sparkling water, may release gas into the stomach, raising pressure and perhaps causing the LES to relax.

Explanation of Why Some Foods Can Be Harmful:

1. Acidity Levels:

• Acidic foods, such as citrus fruits and tomatoes, can directly contribute to increased stomach acid, causing esophageal discomfort.

2. LES Relaxation:

• Many trigger foods, including chocolate, mint, onions, garlic, and spicy foods, can relax the lower esophageal sphincter. Stomach acid is more prone to reflux into the esophagus when the LES is not securely closed.

3. High Fat Content:

• Fatty foods take longer to digest, causing the stomach to feel fuller for longer periods. This can increase pressure on the LES and cause stomach emptying to be delayed, causing acid reflux.

4. Caffeine:

• Caffeine, present in coffee, tea, and some sodas, is known to relax the LES, allowing stomach acid to flow back into the esophagus more easily.

5. Alcohol and Carbonation:

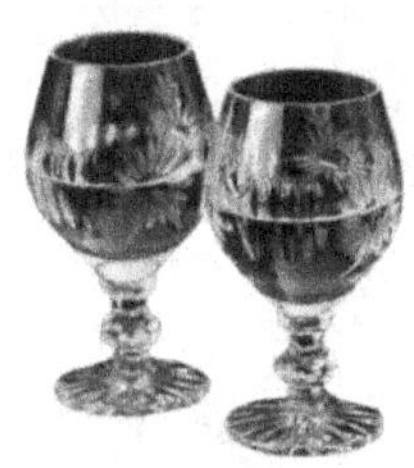
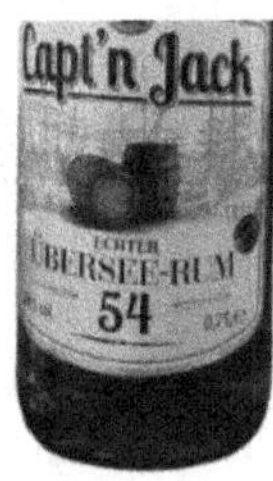

• Both alcohol and carbonated drinks can relax the LES while also increasing stomach acid production. Furthermore, carbonated beverages can transfer gas into the stomach, causing pressure and perhaps contributing to acid reflux.

Understanding the effects of different foods on acid reflux and making smart dietary choices are crucial for managing and preventing symptoms. Individuals can lessen the frequency and intensity of acid reflux episodes by avoiding trigger foods and implementing lifestyle changes that support improved digestive health.

CHAPTER 6: FOODS TO EMBRACE

In order to reverse acid reflux and promote a healthier digestive system, you must incorporate specific foods into your diet that can help calm and prevent acid reflux symptoms. A well-balanced and healthy diet is essential for overall digestive health.

Here are key points to consider:

Foods to Eat to Reverse Acid Reflux:

Ginger:

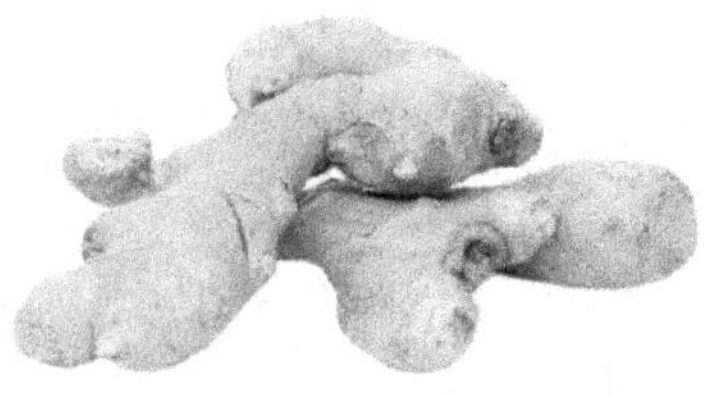

Ginger contains anti-inflammatory qualities that can calm the esophagus and alleviate acid reflux symptoms. It may be consumed in a variety of ways, such as ginger tea or by adding it to meals.

OATMEAL:

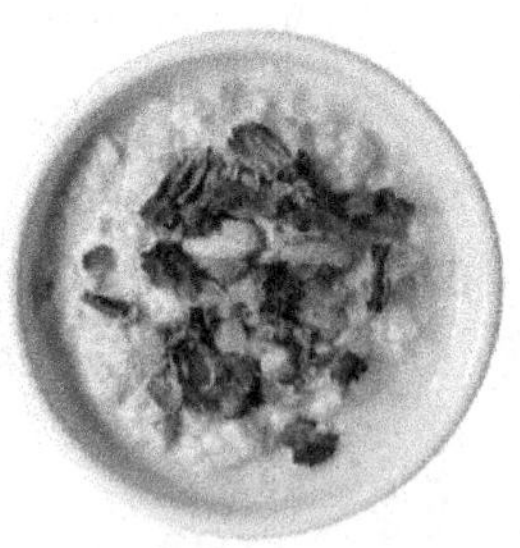

Oatmeal is a complete grain that can absorb excess stomach acid and soothe the esophagus. For the greatest results, use plain, unflavored oatmeal.

Fruits That Are Not Citrus:

While citrus fruits are frequent triggers, non-citrus alternatives such as bananas, melons, apples, and pears are typically well-tolerated and can help relieve acid reflux symptoms.

Vegetables:

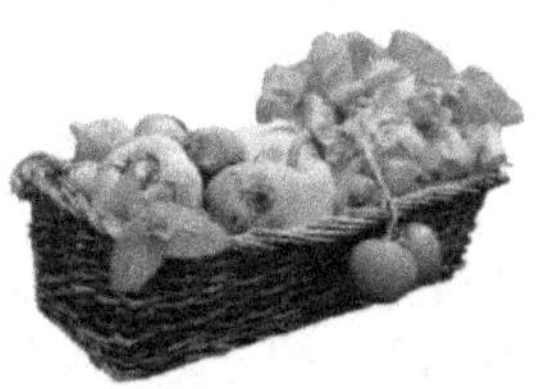

Most vegetables, particularly leafy greens such as kale and spinach, are low in acidity and can help to maintain a healthy, well-balanced diet. However, tomatoes and other extremely acidic foods should be avoided.

Proteins That Are Low In Fat:

Choose lean protein sources including chicken, turkey, fish, and tofu. These proteins are easier to digest and are less susceptible to triggering excessive acid production.

Whole Grain:

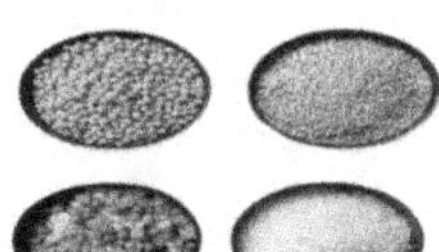

Whole grains, such as brown rice, quinoa, and whole wheat bread, are high in fiber and can help with digestion. They also aid in the absorption of stomach acid, lowering the risk of reflux.

Milk from Almonds:

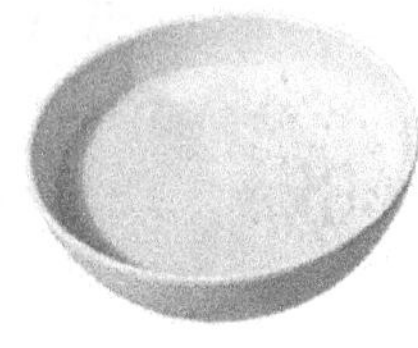

Almond milk is a non-acidic alternative to ordinary dairy milk that can be calming to people who suffer from acid reflux. To eliminate extra sugars, use an unsweetened kind.

Herbal Teas:

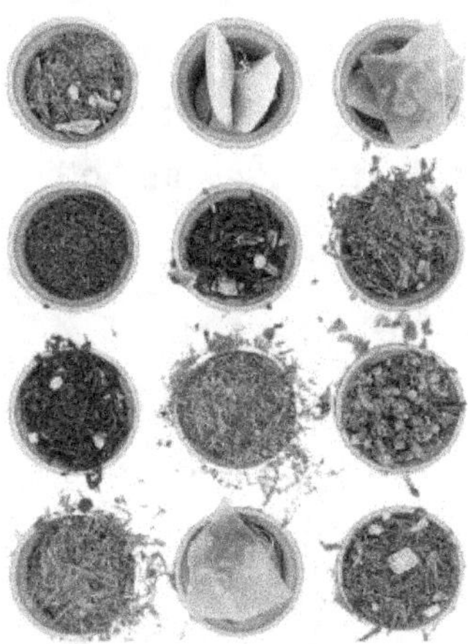

The anti-inflammatory properties of chamomile and licorice root tea can help relax the digestive tract. They can be utilized between meals to provide further relief.

Aloe Vera Juice:

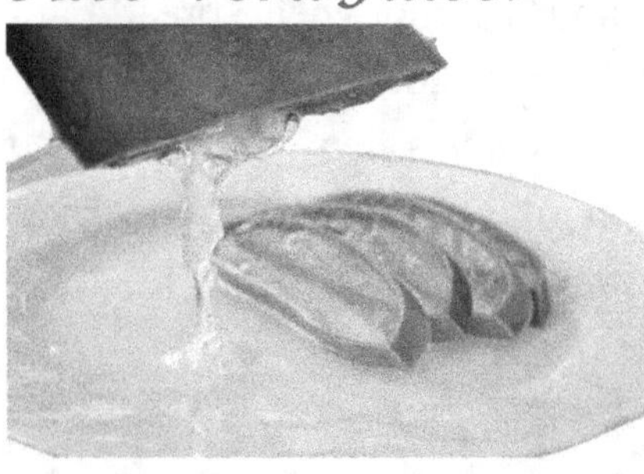

Aloe vera juice may be soothing to the esophagus and aid in the reduction of inflammation. It is crucial to select aloe vera juice that has been carefully prepared for internal usage.

The Importance of a Well-balanced and Nutritious Diet:

Keeping a Healthy Weight:

A healthy diet promotes weight control, which is essential for limiting stomach pressure and lowering the risk of acid reflux.

Foods High in Fiber:

Fiber encourages regular bowel movements and aids in the prevention of constipation, which can aggravate acid reflux. Complete grains, fruits, and vegetables are rich in fiber.

Overeating Prevention:

Consuming smaller, more frequent meals rather than larger ones helps to avoid stomach overburden and reduces the likelihood of acid reflux.

Hydration:

Drinking enough water throughout the day aids digestion and helps to preserve the mucosal lining of the esophagus.

Limiting the Consumption of Processed Foods:

Highly processed and oily foods could worsen acid reflux symptoms by contributing to inflammation. A concentration of whole, unprocessed foods is helpful.

Macronutrient Balance:

A well-balanced diet has a variety of carbs, proteins, and healthy fats. Keeping excesses in any macronutrient group to a minimum promotes intestinal health.

Finally, a diet rich in calming and acid reflux-friendly foods is essential for reversing symptoms and creating a healthier digestive tract. A well-balanced and healthy diet, together with lifestyle changes, contributes to long-term digestive health. Adopting whole foods, keeping a healthy weight, and paying attention to portion sizes are all important steps in the quest to relieve and prevent acid reflux.

IV. Acid Reflux Reversal Recipes

CHAPTER 7: BREAKFAST BLISS

Here are 10 acid-reflux-friendly breakfast recipes with detailed ingredients, preparation methods, quantity, nutritional value, and cooking time:

1. *Oatmeal with Bananas and Almonds:*

- **Ingredients:**

- 1/2 cup rolled oats

- 1 cup almond milk

- 1 ripe banana, sliced

- 1 tablespoon sliced almonds

- Nutritional Value:

- Fiber-rich oats for digestion, potassium from bananas, and healthy fats from almonds.

- Cooking Time:

- 5 minutes

- **Preparation:**

Follow the package instructions in cooking the oats with almond milk.

Top with banana slices and sliced almonds.

Stir gently and enjoy!

2. *Greek Yogurt Parfait:*

- **Ingredients:**

- 1/2 cup Greek yogurt

- 1/4 cup granola (low-fat)

- 1/4 cup mixed berries (blueberries, strawberries)

- **Nutritional Value:**

- Protein from Greek yogurt, fiber from granola, and antioxidants from berries.

- **Cooking Time:**

- 5 minutes

- **Preparation:**

Layer the Greek yogurt, granola, and mixed berries in a glass.

Repeat the layers.

Finish with a drizzle of honey if desired.

3. *Egg White Veggie Omelette:*

- **Ingredients:**

- 3 egg whites

- 1/4 cup bell peppers (diced)

- 1/4 cup spinach (chopped)

- 1 tablespoon feta cheese (optional)

- **Nutritional Value:**

- High protein from egg whites, vitamins from veggies, and calcium from feta.

- **Cooking Time:**

- 10 minutes

- **Preparation:**

Whisk the egg whites in a bowl.

Pour into a preheated, non-stick pan.

Add bell peppers, spinach, and feta cheese.

Fold the omelet and cook until set.

4. *Whole Grain Toast with Avocado:*

- **Ingredients:**

- 2 slices whole grain bread

- 1/2 avocado, mashed

- Pinch of salt and pepper

- **Nutritional Value:**

- Fiber from whole grain bread and healthy fats from avocado.

- **Cooking Time:**

- 5 minutes

- **Preparation:**

- Toast bread, spread mashed avocado, and season.

5. *Chia Seed Pudding:*

- **Ingredients:**

- 2 tablespoons chia seeds

- 1/2 cup almond milk

- 1/4 teaspoon vanilla extract

- 1 teaspoon honey

- **Nutritional Value:**

- Omega-3 fatty acids from chia seeds, calcium from almond milk.

- **Preparation:**

In a bowl, mix chia seeds, almond milk, vanilla extract, and honey.

Stir well and refrigerate overnight.

Top with your favorite berries before serving.

6. Smoothie Bowl:

- **Ingredients:**

- 1/2 cup plain yogurt

- 1/2 cup mixed berries

- 1/2 banana, sliced

- 1 tablespoon honey

- **Nutritional Value:**

- Probiotics from yogurt, antioxidants from berries, and potassium from bananas.

- **Cooking Time:**

- 5 minutes

- **Preparation:**

Blend yogurt and mixed berries until smooth.

Pour the smoothie into a bowl.

Top with banana slices and drizzle with honey.

7. Quinoa Breakfast Bowl:

- **Ingredients:**

- 1/2 cup cooked quinoa

- 1/4 cup sliced almonds

- 1/4 cup dried cranberries

- 1/2 teaspoon cinnamon

- **Nutritional Value:**

- Protein from quinoa, healthy fats from almonds, and antioxidants from cranberries.

- **Cooking Time:**

- 15 minutes (including quinoa preparation)

- **Preparation:**

In a bowl, mix cooked quinoa, sliced almonds, dried cranberries, and cinnamon.

Adjust sweetness to taste.

8. *Baked Apples with Cinnamon:*

- **Ingredients:**

- 2 apples, cored and sliced

- 1/2 teaspoon cinnamon

- 1 tablespoon maple syrup (optional)

- **Nutritional Value:**

- Fiber from apples and anti-inflammatory properties of cinnamon.

- **Cooking Time:**

- 20 minutes

- **Preparation:**

Preheat the oven to 375°F (190°C).

Toss apple slices with cinnamon and optional maple syrup.

Bake for 20 minutes or until tender.

9. *Brown Rice Porridge:*

- **Ingredients:**

- 1/2 cup cooked brown rice

- 1/2 cup almond milk

- 1 tablespoon raisins

- 1/4 teaspoon nutmeg

- **Nutritional Value:**

- Fiber from brown rice, calcium from almond milk, and natural sweetness from raisins.

- **Cooking Time:**

- 10 minutes

- **Preparation:**

In a saucepan, heat brown rice with almond milk.

Stir in raisins and nutmeg.

Simmer until heated through.

10.   *Cottage Cheese with Pineapple:*

- **Ingredients:**

- 1/2 cup low-fat cottage cheese

- 1/2 cup pineapple chunks

- 1 tablespoon chopped mint (optional)

- **Nutritional Value:**

- Protein from cottage cheese and digestive enzymes from pineapple.

- **Cooking Time:**

- 5 minutes

- **Preparation:**

Combine cottage cheese and pineapple chunks.

Garnish with chopped mint if desired.

Enjoy this refreshing and protein-packed breakfast!

These breakfast recipes are easy to prepare and include a range of flavors that are friendly to acid reflux. Adjust the ingredients and quantities to suit your tastes and dietary requirements.

These breakfast dishes are not only acid reflux-friendly, but also high in nutrients to help you start your day off right. Portion sizes should be adjusted based on individual nutritional needs and preferences.

CHAPTER 8: DELECTABLE LUNCHES

Here are ten acid-reflux-friendly lunch dishes with complete ingredient lists, preparation techniques, serving sizes, nutritional value, and cooking times:

1. *Grilled Chicken Salad:*

- **Ingredients:**

- 4 oz boneless, skinless chicken breast

- 2 cups mixed greens (lettuce, spinach)

- 1/2 cucumber, sliced

- 1/2 cup cherry tomatoes, halved

- 1 tablespoon olive oil

- **Nutritional Value:**

- Lean protein from chicken, fiber from vegetables, and healthy fats from olive oil.

- **Cooking Time:**

- 15 minutes (including grilling)

- **Preparation:**

Season chicken breast with salt and pepper.

Cook through grilling (about 6 – 8 minutes per side).

Slice the grilled chicken.

In a bowl, combine mixed greens, cucumber, cherry tomatoes, and sliced grilled chicken.

Drizzle with olive oil and toss gently.

2. *Quinoa and Vegetable Stir-Fry:*

- **Ingredients:**

- 1/2 cup cooked quinoa

- 1 cup mixed vegetables (broccoli, bell peppers, snap peas)

- 2 tablespoons low-sodium soy sauce

- 1 tablespoon sesame oil

- **Nutritional Value:**

- Protein and fiber from quinoa, vitamins from vegetables, and healthy fats from sesame oil.

- **Cooking Time:**

- 15 minutes

- **Preparation:**

- In a pan, heat sesame oil over medium heat.

- Add mixed vegetables and stir-fry until tender-crisp.

- Add cooked quinoa and soy sauce, and toss until well combined.

- Serve hot.

3. *Salmon with Roasted Vegetables:*

- **Ingredients:**

- 4 oz salmon fillet

- 1 cup mixed vegetables (zucchini, cherry tomatoes, bell peppers)

- 1 tablespoon olive oil

- 1/2 teaspoon dried herbs (rosemary, thyme)

- **Nutritional Value:**

- Omega-3 fatty acids from salmon, fiber from vegetables, and anti-inflammatory properties from herbs.

- **Cooking Time:**

- 20 minutes (including roasting)

Preparation:

Preheat the oven to 400°F (200°C).

Place salmon on a baking sheet, and surround it with mixed vegetables.

Drizzle olive oil over the salmon and vegetables.

Sprinkle dried herbs.

Roast for 15-20 minutes or until salmon is cooked through.

4. *Turkey and Avocado Wrap:*

- **Ingredients**:

- 4 oz lean turkey slices

- 1 whole-grain wrap

- 1/2 avocado, sliced

- 1 cup mixed greens

- **Nutritional Value:**

- Lean protein from turkey, fiber from the wrap, and healthy fats from avocado.

- **Preparation Time:**

- 10 minutes

- **Preparation:**

Lay the whole-grain wrap flat.

Arrange turkey slices, avocado slices, and mixed greens.

Wrap up the roll tightly and slice it into two halves.

5. *Vegetarian Lentil Soup:*

- **Ingredients:**

- 1/2 cup dry lentils

- 1 carrot, diced

- 1 celery stalk, diced

- 1/2 onion, chopped

- 1 clove garlic, minced

- 4 cups vegetable broth

- **Nutritional Value:**

- Protein and fiber from lentils, vitamins from vegetables, and low-fat content.

- **Cooking Time:**

- 30 minutes

- **Preparation:**

Sauté the onion and garlic in a pot until they become soft.

Add lentils, carrots, celery, and vegetable broth.

Allow it to simmer for 25-30 minutes or until the lentils are tender.

6. *Egg and Spinach Stuffed Sweet Potato:*

- **Ingredients:**

- 1 medium sweet potato

- 2 eggs

- 1 cup fresh spinach

- Salt and pepper to taste

- **Nutritional Value:**

- Fiber from sweet potato, protein from eggs, and vitamins from spinach.

- **Cooking Time:**

- 45 minutes (including baking sweet potato)

- **Preparation:**

Preheat the oven to 400°F (200°C).

Bake the sweet potato for 40-45 minutes until tender.

Cut a slit in the sweet potato and fluff the insides with a fork.

In a pan, wilt spinach.

Crack eggs into the pan and scramble until cooked.

Stuff the sweet potato with the spinach and scrambled eggs.

Season with salt and pepper.

7. Shrimp and Quinoa Bowl:

- **Ingredients:**

- 4 oz shrimp, peeled and deveined

- 1/2 cup cooked quinoa

- 1 cup steamed broccoli

- 1 tablespoon olive oil

- **Nutritional Value:**

- Protein from shrimp, fiber from quinoa, and vitamins from broccoli.

- **Cooking Time:**

- 15 minutes

- **Preparation:**

Heat the olive oil in a pan over medium heat.

Add shrimp and cook until pink and opaque.

Assemble the bowl with cooked quinoa, steamed broccoli, and cooked shrimp.

8. *Baked Chicken with Asparagus:*

- **Ingredients:**

- 4 oz chicken breast

- 1 bunch asparagus, trimmed

- 1 tablespoon lemon juice

- 1 teaspoon dried oregano

- **Nutritional Value:**

- Lean protein from chicken, fiber from asparagus, and anti-inflammatory properties from lemon and oregano.

- **Cooking Time:**

- 25 minutes (including baking)

- **Preparation**

Preheat the oven to 375°F (190°C).

Place chicken breast on a baking sheet.

Arrange asparagus around the chicken.

Drizzle with lemon juice and sprinkle with dried oregano.

Bake for 20-25 minutes or until chicken is cooked through.

9. *Brown Rice and Vegetable Bowl:*

- **Ingredients:**

- 1/2 cup cooked brown rice

- 1/2 cup mixed vegetables (bell peppers, carrots, snap peas)

- 2 tablespoons low-sodium teriyaki sauce

- 1 tablespoon chopped green onions

- **Nutritional Value:**

- Fiber from brown rice, vitamins from vegetables, and low-sodium teriyaki for flavor.

- Cooking Time:

- 15 minutes

- **Preparation:**

In a pan, sauté mixed vegetables until tender.

Add cooked brown rice and teriyaki sauce, and toss until well coated.

Garnish with chopped green onions.

10. *Mediterranean Chickpea Salad:*

- **Ingredients:**

  - 1 can (15 oz) chickpeas, drained and rinsed

  - 1 cucumber, diced

  - 1 cup cherry tomatoes, halved

  - 1/4 cup feta cheese, crumbled

  - 2 tablespoons olive oil

- **Nutritional Value:**

  - Protein and fiber from chickpeas, vitamins from vegetables, and healthy fats from olive oil.

  - Preparation Time:

  - 10 minutes

- **Preparation:**

In a bowl, combine chickpeas, cucumber, cherry tomatoes, and feta cheese.

Drizzle with olive oil and toss gently.

Serve chilled.

These lunch recipes are not only acid reflux-friendly but also provide a balance of nutrients for a well-rounded and satisfying meal. Adjust portion sizes based on individual dietary needs and preferences.

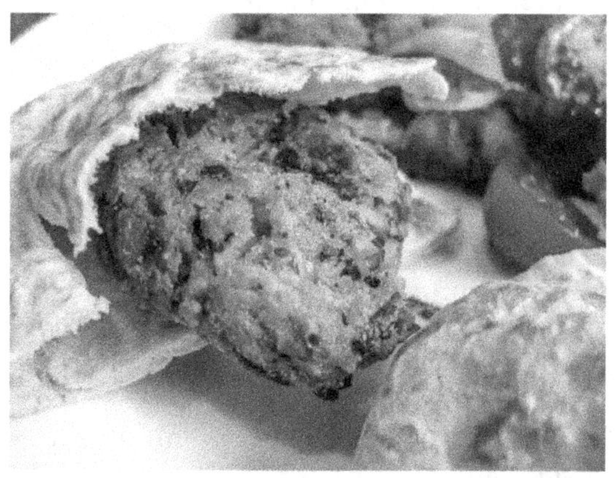

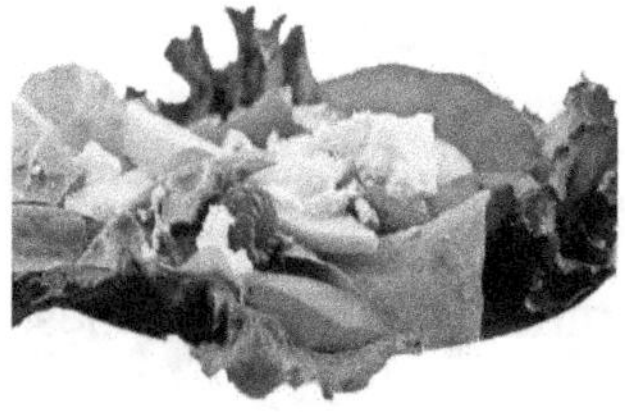

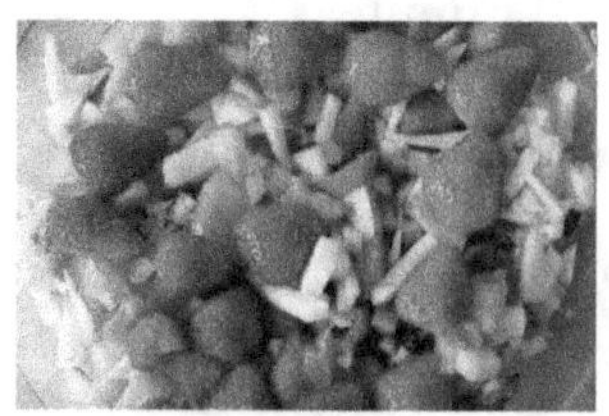

Here are 10 acid-reflux-friendly dinner recipes with detailed ingredients, preparation instructions, quantity, nutritional value, and cooking time:

1. *Baked Cod with Lemon and Herbs:*

- **Ingredients:**

- 4 oz cod fillet

- 1 tablespoon olive oil

- 1 tablespoon lemon juice

- 1 teaspoon dried herbs (such as thyme or dill)

- **Nutritional Value:**

- Lean protein from cod, anti-inflammatory properties from lemon and herbs.

- **Cooking Time:**

- 20 minutes (including baking)

•**Preparation:**

Preheat the oven to 375°F (190°C).

Place the cod fillet on a baking sheet.

Drizzle with olive oil and lemon juice.

Sprinkle dried herbs over the cod.

Bake for 15-20 minutes or until the cod flakes easily with a fork.

2. *Vegetable and Chickpea Stir-Fry:*

- **Ingredients:**

- 1 cup mixed vegetables (bell peppers, broccoli, carrots)

- 1 can (15 oz) chickpeas, drained and rinsed

- 2 tablespoons low-sodium soy sauce

- 1 tablespoon sesame oil

- **Nutritional Value:**

- Protein and fiber from chickpeas, vitamins from vegetables, and healthy fats from sesame oil.

- **Cooking Time:**

- 15 minutes

- **Preparation:**

Heat the sesame oil in a large pan over medium heat.

Add mixed vegetables and stir-fry until crisp-tender.

Add chickpeas and soy sauce, and stir until heated through.

Dish out the meal over a bed of quinoa or brown rice.

3. *Turkey and Quinoa Stuffed Bell Peppers:*

- **Ingredients:**

- 1/2 cup cooked quinoa

- 4 oz ground turkey

- 2 bell peppers, halved

- 1/2 cup tomato sauce (low-acid)

- **Nutritional Value:**

- Protein from turkey, fiber from quinoa, and vitamins from bell peppers.

- **Cooking Time:**

- 30 minutes (including baking)

- **Preparation:**

Preheat the oven to 375°F (190°C).

In a skillet, cook ground turkey until browned.

Mix cooked quinoa with browned turkey.

Fill bell pepper halves with the quinoa and turkey mixture.

Top with tomato sauce.

Bake for 20-25 minutes.

4. *Salmon and Asparagus Foil Packets:*

- **Ingredients:**

- 4 oz salmon fillet

- 1 bunch asparagus, trimmed

- 1 tablespoon olive oil

- 1 lemon, sliced

- **Nutritional Value:**

- Omega-3 fatty acids from salmon, fiber from asparagus, and anti-inflammatory properties from olive oil and lemon.

- **Cooking Time:**

- 20 minutes (including baking)

- **Preparation:**

Preheat the oven to 400°F (200°C).

Put each salmon fillet on top of a piece of foil

Arrange asparagus around the salmon.

Use olive oil to drizzle over the salmon and asparagus

Place lemon slices on top.

Seal the foil packets and bake for 15-20 minutes.

5. *Cauliflower Rice Bowl with Tofu:*

- **Ingredients:**

- 1 cup cauliflower rice

- 4 oz firm tofu, cubed

- 1 cup of a mixture of vegetables (zucchini, bell peppers)

- 1 tablespoon low-sodium soy sauce

- **Nutritional Value:**

- Protein from tofu, vitamins from vegetables, and low-carb alternative with cauliflower rice.

- **Cooking Time:**

- 15 minutes

- **Preparation:**

In a pan, sauté tofu until golden brown.

Add mixed vegetables and cook until tender.

Stir in cauliflower rice and soy sauce.

Cook until heated through.

6. *Quinoa and Black Bean Salad:*

- **Ingredients:**

- 1/2 cup cooked quinoa

- 1 can (15 oz) of black beans that has been drained and rinsed

- 1 cup cherry tomatoes, halved

- 2 tablespoons olive oil

- **Nutritional Value:**

- Protein and fiber from quinoa and black beans, vitamins from tomatoes, and healthy fats from olive oil.

- **Preparation Time:**

- 10 minutes

- **Preparation:**

In a large bowl, combine quinoa, black beans, and cherry tomatoes.

Drizzle with olive oil and toss gently.

Chill before serving.

7. *Chicken and Broccoli Stir-Fry:*

- **Ingredients:**

- 4 oz chicken breast, sliced

- 1 cup broccoli florets

- 1 tablespoon low-sodium soy sauce

- 1 teaspoon sesame oil

- **Nutritional Value:**

- Lean protein from chicken, vitamins from broccoli, and healthy fats from sesame oil.

- **Cooking Time:**

- 15 minutes

. **Preparation:**

In a wok or large pan, heat sesame oil over medium heat.

Add sliced chicken and stir-fry until cooked through.

Add broccoli and soy sauce, and continue to stir-fry until broccoli is crisp-tender.

Serve over brown rice or quinoa

8. *Eggplant and Lentil Curry:*

- **Ingredients:**

- 1 cup eggplant, diced

- 1/2 cup dry lentils

- 1 can (14 oz) coconut milk (unsweetened)

- 2 tablespoons curry powder

- **Nutritional Value:**

- Fiber from eggplant and lentils, protein from lentils, and healthy fats from coconut milk.

- **Cooking Time:**

- 30 minutes

.   **Preparation:**

In a pot, combine lentils, diced eggplant, coconut milk, and curry powder.

Bring to a simmer and cook for 25-30 minutes or until lentils are tender.

9. *Spinach and Turkey Meatballs:*

- **Ingredients:**

- 4 oz ground turkey

- 1 cup fresh spinach, chopped

- 1/4 cup breadcrumbs (whole wheat)

- 1/4 cup grated Parmesan cheese

- **Nutritional Value:**

- Lean protein from turkey, vitamins from spinach, and calcium from Parmesan cheese.

- **Cooking Time:**

- 20 minutes (including baking)

.   **Preparation:**

Preheat the oven to 375°F (190°C).

In a bowl, combine ground turkey, chopped spinach, breadcrumbs, and Parmesan cheese.

Shape into meatballs and bake for 15-20 minutes.

Mushroom and Spinach Stuffed

10.   *Mushroom and Spinach Stuffed Chicken Breast:*

- **Ingredients:**

- 4 oz chicken breast

- 1/2 cup mushrooms, chopped

- 1 cup fresh spinach

- 1 tablespoon olive oil

- **Nutritional Value:**

- Lean protein from chicken, vitamins from spinach, and anti-inflammatory properties from olive oil.

- **Cooking Time:**

- 25 minutes (including baking)

- **Preparation:**

Preheat the oven to 375°F (190°C).

In a bowl, combine ground turkey, chopped spinach, breadcrumbs, and Parmesan cheese.

Shape into meatballs and bake for 15-20 minutes.

These dinner recipes are not only acid reflux-friendly but also offer a variety of flavors and nutrients for a well-rounded and satisfying evening meal. Adapt portion quantities based on individual's dietary requirements and preferences.

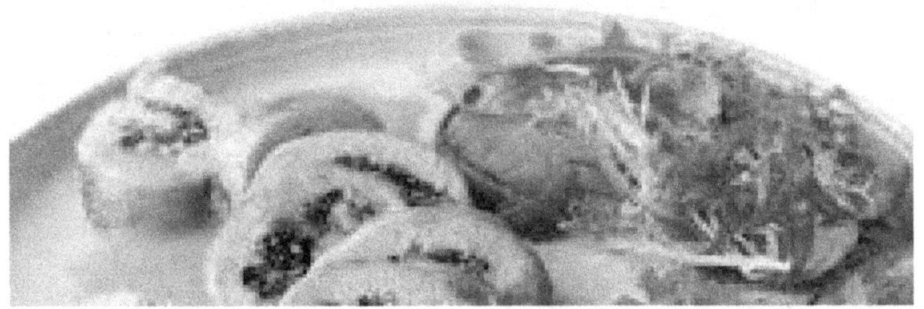

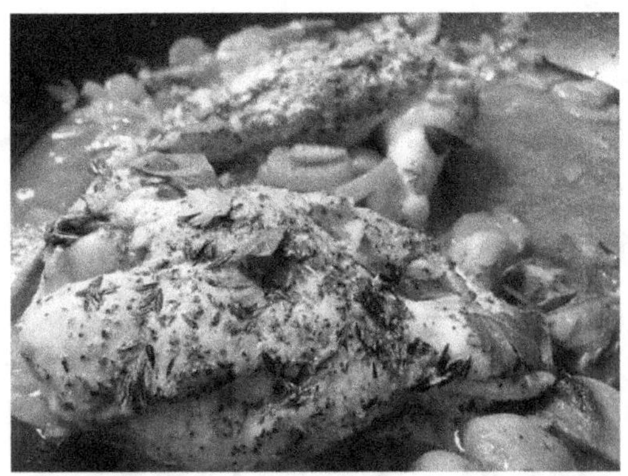

CHAPTER 10: SNACKS AND DESSERTS

Here are 10 acid reflux-friendly snacks and 10 desserts that are suitable for on-the-go consumption, designed to curb hunger without causing discomfort:

Snacks:

1. *Almond and Dried Fruit Mix:*

- **Ingredients:**

- Almonds

- Dried apricots

- Dried cranberries

- **Preparation:**

- Mix almonds with dried apricots and cranberries for a satisfying and portable snack.

2. *Greek Yogurt with Berries:*

- **Ingredients:**

- Plain Greek yogurt

- Mixed berries (blueberries, raspberries)

- **Preparation:**

- Pack a small container with Greek yogurt and top with fresh berries.

3. *Cucumber and Hummus Slices:*

- **Ingredients:**

- Cucumber slices

- Hummus

- **Preparation:**

- Carry cucumber slices and a small container of hummus for a crunchy and satisfying snack.

4. *Rice Cake with Almond Butter:*

- **Ingredients:**

- Brown rice cake

- Almond butter

- **Preparation:**

- Spread almond butter on a rice cake for a quick and portable energy boost.

5. *Apple Slices with Peanut Butter:*

- **Ingredients:**

- Apple slices

- Natural peanut butter

- **Preparation:**

- Dip apple slices into peanut butter for a balanced and delicious snack.

6.   *Oat and Banana Muffins*:

- **Ingredients:**

- Oat flour muffins

- Banana slices

- **Preparation:**

- Bake oat flour muffins with ripe banana slices for a light and portable treat.

7.   *Carrot Sticks with Hummus:*

- **Ingredients:**

- Carrot sticks

- Hummus

- **Preparation:**

- Pair carrot sticks with hummus for a crunchy and satisfying on-the-go snack.

8.   *Trail Mix with Seeds:*

- **Ingredients:**

- Mixed nuts

- Pumpkin seeds

- Sunflower seeds

- **Preparation:**

- Create a trail mix with assorted nuts and seeds for a protein-packed snack.

9. *Cheese and Whole Grain Crackers:*

- **Ingredients:**

- Cheese slices

- Whole grain crackers

- **Preparation:**

- Combine cheese and whole grain crackers for a portable and balanced snack.

10. *Dark Chocolate Covered Almonds:*

- **Ingredients:**

- Dark chocolate-covered almonds

- **Preparation:**

- Purchase pre-made dark chocolate-covered almonds for a sweet and satisfying treat.

Desserts:

1. *Banana and Walnut Oat Bars:*

- **Ingredients:**

- Banana and walnut oat bars

- **Preparation:**
- Bake or purchase banana and walnut oat bars for a wholesome dessert.

2. *Chia Seed Pudding with Berries:*

- **Ingredients:**
- Chia seed pudding
- Mixed berries
- **Preparation:**
- Layer chia seed pudding with mixed berries for a tasty and portable dessert.

3. *Coconut Yogurt Parfait:*

- **Ingredients:**
- Coconut yogurt
- Granola (low-fat)
- Sliced strawberries
- **Preparation:**
- Assemble a parfait with coconut yogurt, low-fat granola, and sliced strawberries.

4. *Frozen Grapes:*

- **Ingredients:**
- Frozen grapes

- **Preparation:**

- Freeze grapes for a refreshing and natural sweet treat.

5. *Peach and Almond Smoothie:*

- **Ingredients:**

- Peach and almond smoothie

- **Preparation:**

- Blend a peach and almond smoothie for a creamy and nutritious dessert.

6. *Vanilla Chia Pudding:*

- **Ingredients:**

- Vanilla chia pudding

- **Preparation:**

- Enjoy a serving of vanilla chia pudding for a satisfying and guilt-free dessert.

7. *Baked Apple Slices with Cinnamon:*

- **Ingredients:**

- Baked apple slices

- Cinnamon

- **Preparation:**

- Bake apple slices with a sprinkle of cinnamon for a warm and comforting dessert.

8. *Mango Sorbet:*

- **Ingredients:**

- Mango sorbet

- **Preparation:**

- Go for mango sorbet as a cool and fruity dessert option.

9. *Blueberry and Oat Cookies:*

- **Ingredients:**

- Blueberry and oat cookies

- **Preparation:**

- Bake or purchase blueberry and oat cookies for a wholesome treat.

10. *Pineapple and Mint Infused Water:*

- **Ingredients:**

- Pineapple and mint-infused water

- **Preparation:**

- Infuse water with pineapple and mint for a refreshing and hydrating dessert alternative.

These snacks and desserts are not only convenient for on-the-go consumption but also mindful of acid reflux triggers. Adjust ingredients and quantities based on personal preferences and dietary needs.

V.   Meal Plans

CHAPTER 11: MEAL PLANNING

- Meal Planning for Acid Reflux Reversal Diet: Benefits and Key Practices

Food Selection:

- Choose foods less likely to trigger acid reflux, such as lean proteins, whole grains, fruits, and vegetables.

- Avoid known triggers like citrus fruits, tomatoes, and spicy foods.

Portion Control:

- Practice careful portion control to prevent overeating.

- Reduce pressure on the lower esophageal sphincter (LES) to minimize acid reflux symptoms.

Timing and Spacing:

- Space meals throughout the day to aid digestion.

- Avoid large, heavy meals close to bedtime to reduce the risk of nighttime acid reflux.

Nutrient-Dense Choices:

- Incorporate a variety of nutrient-dense foods into the diet.

- Ensure a well-balanced intake of essential vitamins and minerals for overall health.

- *Proactive Strategy:*

- Empower individuals to take control of their diet through informed choices.

- Work towards the effective management and potential reversal of acid reflux symptoms.

Meal planning serves as a structured approach, helping individuals make dietary decisions that align to manage and reverse acid reflux.

WEEKLY MEAL PLAN

Here's a sample 7-day meal plan for acid reflux reversal, including breakfast, lunch, and dinner:

Day 1:
Breakfast:
Oatmeal with sliced bananas and a sprinkle of almonds.

Herbal tea.

Lunch:
Grilled chicken salad with mixed greens, cucumber, and cherry tomatoes.

Olive oil and lemon dressing.

Dinner:

Baked cod with lemon and herbs.

Quinoa and steamed broccoli on the side.

Day 2:
Breakfast:

Greek yogurt parfait with low-fat granola and mixed berries.

Lunch:

Turkey and avocado wrap with whole-grain tortilla.

Mixed green salad.

Dinner:

Quinoa and vegetable stir-fry with tofu.

Brown rice on the side.

Day 3:
Breakfast:

Egg white veggie omelette with bell peppers and spinach.

Whole grain toast.

Lunch:

Salmon with roasted vegetables (zucchini, cherry tomatoes).

Olive oil and herbs for flavor.

Dinner:

Mediterranean chickpea salad with diced cucumber and cherry tomatoes.

Day 4:
Breakfast:

Chia seed pudding with almond milk, topped with fresh berries.

Lunch:

Vegetarian lentil soup with diced carrots and celery.

Dinner:

Turkey and quinoa stuffed bell peppers with a side of tomato sauce.

Day 5:
Breakfast:

Smoothie bowl with plain yogurt, mixed berries, banana slices, and honey drizzle.

Lunch:

Egg and spinach stuffed sweet potato.

Dinner:

Baked chicken with asparagus, drizzled with lemon juice.

Day 6:

Breakfast:

Cottage cheese with pineapple chunks and a touch of chopped mint.

Lunch:

Shrimp and quinoa bowl with steamed broccoli.

Dinner:

Quinoa and black bean salad with cherry tomatoes.

Day 7:

Breakfast:

Brown rice porridge with almond milk, raisins, and a hint of nutmeg.

Lunch:

Mushroom and spinach stuffed chicken breast.

Dinner:

Cauliflower rice bowl with tofu and mixed vegetables.

Adjust portion sizes based on individual needs and preferences. It's important to stay hydrated throughout the day, and for snacks, consider options like fresh fruit, nuts, or yogurt. This meal plan focuses on nutrient-dense, non-triggering foods to support acid reflux reversal.

BONUS

BONUS 1: 4 WEEKS WEEKLY MEAL PLANNER

Weekly Meal Planner

	Breakfast	Lunch	Dinner	Snack
Sunday				
Monday				
Tuesday				
Wednesday				
Thursday				
Friday				
Saturday				

Shopping List:

Weekly Meal Planner

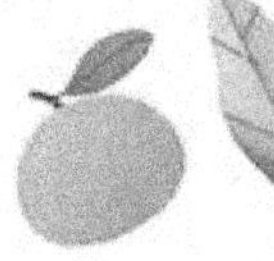

	Breakfast	Lunch	Dinner	Snack
Sunday				
Monday				
Tuesday				
Wednesday				
Thursday				
Friday				
Saturday				

Shopping List :

Weekly Meal Planner

	Breakfast	Lunch	Dinner	Snack
Sunday				
Monday				
Tuesday				
Wednesday				
Thursday				
Friday				
Saturday				

Shopping List :

BONUS 2: HOURLY-DAILY-WEEKLY MEAL MONITORING SCHEDULE

WEEKLY SCHEDULE

TIME	MONDAY	TUESDAY	WEDNESDAY	THURSDAY	FRIDAY	SATURDAY	SUNDAY
7 AM							
8 AM							
9 AM							
10 AM							
11 AM							
12 PM							
1 PM							
2 PM							
3 PM							
4 PM							
5 PM							
6 PM							
7 PM							
8 PM							
9 PM							
10 PM							

WEEKLY SCHEDULE

TIME	MONDAY	TUESDAY	WEDNESDAY	THURSDAY	FRIDAY	SATURDAY	SUNDAY
7 AM							
8 AM							
9 AM							
10 AM							
11 AM							
12 PM							
1 PM							
2 PM							
3 PM							
4 PM							
5 PM							
6 PM							
7 PM							
8 PM							
9 PM							
10 PM							

WEEKLY SCHEDULE

TIME	MONDAY	TUESDAY	WEDNESDAY	THURSDAY	FRIDAY	SATURDAY	SUNDAY
7 AM							
8 AM							
9 AM							
10 AM							
11 AM							
12 PM							
1 PM							
2 PM							
3 PM							
4 PM							
5 PM							
6 PM							
7 PM							
8 PM							
9 PM							
10 PM							

WEEKLY SCHEDULE

TIME	MONDAY	TUESDAY	WEDNESDAY	THURSDAY	FRIDAY	SATURDAY	SUNDAY
7 AM							
8 AM							
9 AM							
10 AM							
11 AM							
12 PM							
1 PM							
2 PM							
3 PM							
4 PM							
5 PM							
6 PM							
7 PM							
8 PM							
9 PM							
10 PM							

WEEKLY SCHEDULE

TIME	MONDAY	TUESDAY	WEDNESDAY	THURSDAY	FRIDAY	SATURDAY	SUNDAY
7 AM							
8 AM							
9 AM							
10 AM							
11 AM							
12 PM							
1 PM							
2 PM							
3 PM							
4 PM							
5 PM							
6 PM							
7 PM							
8 PM							
9 PM							
10 PM							

CONCLUSION

This Acid Reflux Reversal Manual and Cookbook provides a comprehensive and practical guide to managing acid reflux symptoms through a thoughtfully curated collection of delicious and nutritious recipes. The carefully crafted meal plans, encompassing breakfast, lunch, and dinner options for a span of seven days, reflect a commitment to promoting digestive health and minimizing acid reflux triggers.

This cookbook prioritizes the inclusion of foods known for their soothing and anti-inflammatory properties, avoiding common triggers such as acidic fruits, spicy dishes, and heavy, fatty meals. The integration of lean proteins, whole grains, and a variety of fruits and vegetables ensures a well-balanced and nutrient-rich diet that supports overall well-being.

The recipes presented in this cookbook are not just about managing symptoms but are designed with the potential for acid reflux reversal in mind. By adopting these meal plans, individuals can take a proactive step towards long-term relief and improved digestive health.

It is essential to recognize that dietary changes can have a profound impact on one's well-being. Embracing this acid reflux reversal diet is not merely about restriction; it is an empowering choice to prioritize health and reclaim control over one's life. Each recipe is a step towards better digestion, reduced discomfort, and the potential reversal of acid reflux.

As a special motivation, consider this: by embracing and adapting to this diet, you are investing in your health and well-being. You have the opportunity to cultivate a positive relationship with food, nourish your body with wholesome ingredients, and pave the way for a life free from the constraints of acid reflux symptoms. Remember, the journey to better health starts with small, consistent steps, and this cookbook serves as your roadmap to a life of comfort and vitality. Make the choice to prioritize your health today, and let these recipes guide you towards a future filled with flavorful, reflux-friendly meals and the joy of a well-nourished, thriving body.

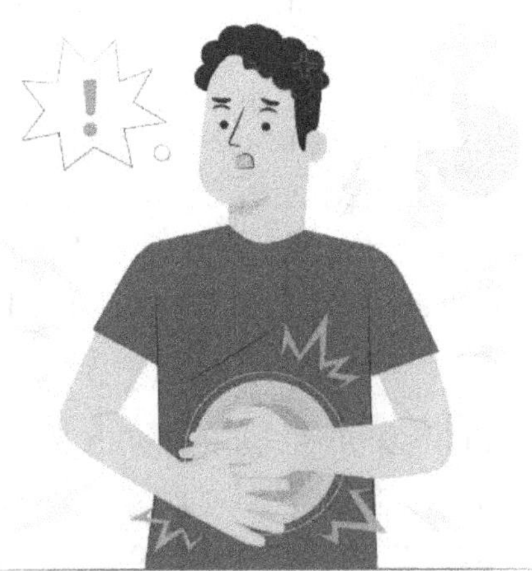

www.ingramcontent.com/pod-product-compliance
Lightning Source LLC
Chambersburg PA
CBHW050833260726
48660CB00006B/2224